Demystifying Stem Cells

A Real Life Approach

By Dr. Bohdan Olesnicky, M.D.

and

Dr. Naota Hashimoto, D.C.

First Edition

ISBN: 978-1530093991

Printed in the United States of America

Table of Contents

Foreword

In 2010, my partner, Dr. Mark Berman, and I used technology brought back from Japan and South Korea to isolate high numbers of viable stem cells from small quantities of liposuction material in the operating room, thus allowing us to transfer millions of healing stem cells from healthy tissue to other parts of the body that were damaged, diseased, or degenerated.

We understood that this gave us an opportunity to provide our patients with regenerative cell therapy on an investigational basis under the auspices of an IRB institutional review board bioethics committee.

This minor surgical procedure, done on an outpatient basis, gave us an opportunity to treat patients with their own stem cells in a completely new way which differed greatly from the traditional pathways used by industry in drug development.

The modern drug industry involves large universities and pharmacology companies who develop products and study them over 10 to 20 year periods. They then patent, bottle and promote them for mass use and commercialization. This is also called monetization.

Our simple surgical stem cell procedure can be done safely and with sterility in any physician's office who has the proper training and equipment. It rapidly became apparent to us that it would be very important for us to teach this procedure to other physicians and help them bring regenerative medicine to the United States and achieve our vision that cell therapy could and should be available in every modern doctor's office.

After having treated thousands of patients and gained experience and knowledge, we have been very fortunate to work with some of the finest physicians in America and help them bring this regenerative technology to their practices and to help their patients heal in a natural way.

We have collected data that shows this procedure appears to be safe and beneficial for a variety of medical conditions. We are very gratified to see high-caliber physicians like Dr. Olesnicky and Dr. Hashimoto collaborating and not only treating patients but also spreading the word providing education to the public through books like *Demystifying Stem Cells*.

Our Cell Surgical Network investigational stem cell technology is now used all over the world and the core model is helping our physicians help their patients and it is an honor to work with very best of the best.

Hopefully readers will learn about this exciting new field through this book and share it with their friends as we propagate the "stem cell revolution."

Elliot B. Lander M.D., F.A.C.S.

Medical Director and Co-Founder of Cell Surgical Network

Introduction

My name is Dr. Bohdan Olesnicky, MD (Dr. O. or, to my friends, Dan O.) and I have written this book with a friend, colleague and business partner Dr. Naota Hashimoto, DC (Dr. H.). We both have come from different but interesting backgrounds and have found a unique synergy in this new field of medicine called Regenerative Medicine.

Being a pioneer in a field is always challenging but sometimes it takes different people with different perspectives coming together with one purpose of delivering the best possible health care so we could help our patients avoid surgery if possible.

I was born in the United States but spent my early childhood in Austria which definitely has a different philosophy of health compared to the United States.

There is definitely less focus on medications and more drive to improve health through lifestyle changes with the goal of minimizing medications and to avoid surgery if possible. The quality of life is stressed as much as the quantity, if not more.

Later in my adult life, I continued to travel and live outside the United States, studying and teaching in various countries. I've treasured my time living in different cultures, learning other languages and being exposed to their approach to health, wellness and medicine.

My pursuit of knowledge started with studies in Archaeology and Physical Anthropology. Later, I pursued Graduate

Introduction

Studies in Molecular Genetics and I seriously considered spending my life in the lab studying stem cells prior to going to Medical School.

My experience with patients as an Emergency Medical Technician (EMT) was what made me decide to follow a more clinical path and become a physician. Never forgetting my research roots, I attended medical school and became a Medical Doctor (MD).

I completed two residencies and became board certified in both Internal Medicine and Emergency Medicine.

I have also lectured internationally on the topic of Tactical Medicine, which is the delivery of medical care and optimal physical performance with Military and Law Enforcement Special Operational Teams.

This dovetailed nicely with the American Academy of Anti-Aging Medicine (A4M).

Currently I hold multiple certifications in Anti-Aging Medicine.

Still as the years have gone on, I have maintained a passion for molecular genetics and stem cells that I studied in graduate school. This is why I was so excited to start as a pioneer in the field of Stem Cells when it became available for human treatment outside of a lab in the clinical setting.

I believe that everything happens for a reason and fate has brought two game changers into my life, Dr. Naota Hashimoto and Dr. Elliot Lander.

I was referred by a colleague to Dr. Hashimoto when I threw out my back and was in need of a good Chiropractor. He was able to fix me up very quickly and we seemed to hit it off immediately.

Over the years we have treated each other, referred to each other and, finally, we started a business together, Desert Medical Care & Wellness, located in La Quinta, CA.

Introduction

Dr. Hashimoto is definitely a unique chiropractor because of his background in physical therapy (in which he has a certificate) and his experience with acupuncture and functional medicine.

He has an amazing practice with more cutting edge equipment for natural pain relief than all of the chiropractors and physical therapists combined in Coachella Valley, California.

He is one of the few chiropractors that consistently receives referrals from physicians because we like the way he practices and he delivers great results.

His treatment is one of my key ingredients to fixing some of our stem cell patients because he corrects the patients structural and alignment problems.

Using stem cells may help repair cartilage, ligaments or tendons but it won't improve the core muscle loss or alignment problem that may have led to your degenerative condition. If you have a pinched nerve, you need to realign the tissues before stem cells can make a real impact.

Our practice together is actually a new field of Medicine called **Integrated Physical Medicine**, which combines the field of medicine with physical treatments like Acupuncture, Chiropractic and Physical Therapy, and allows us to offer the best of both worlds.

This is a great place to receive treatment if you are in pain but still want to avoid surgery.

Dr. Hashimoto even introduced a new therapy to our stem cell protocol that includes using a shockwave device that will drive more blood flow into the affected area and increasing the response from the stem cell therapy. This helps stem cells find their target.

Dr. Lander is the one of the pioneers in this field since 2010 and he introduced me to this stem cell protocol years ago. He is one of the founders of the Cell Surgical Network that I participate in today.

We share case data, protocols and strive to make the experience better for you and all of our patients in the future.

Dr. Lander created the forum where we can share data with other doctors and upload the data about results and protocols that we share with 150+ clinics so we can keep improving our outcomes.

I pride myself on these essential relationships because they have helped me deliver excellent outcomes and I will continue to deliver for years to come. This is why our practice continually receives a constant string of referrals every month that we are in practice.

My core passion is true healthcare (not a sick care system we have today) and hope that this is only the beginning of great things to come in healthcare.

One day, we will be able to heal any disease process, any degenerative joint and eliminate any kind of pain just like Dr. Leonard McCoy did back in Star Trek. We see that the science fiction of yesterday is becoming science fact of today.

My friends will describe me as one of the busiest people they know because my roles include being an ER Doctor, Internal Medicine Doctor, Reserve Police Officer assigned to S.W.A.T., CEO and founder of one of the fastest growing Pro-Line supplement companies called SWAT Fuel, Inc.

From the academic side, I'm an Associate Clinical Professor for Western Medical School and am currently on the Global Protection Medical Group team conducting clinical studies on the Mechanical Blood Volumizer, a lifesaving anti-shock device being taken through the FDA.

Most importantly, I am married to the smartest person I know, Anne Olesnicky,

MD, who is an Anesthesiologist and the Executive Vice President of SWAT Fuel, Inc., all while also the mother to our four children.

I hope that the work I am doing today with stem cells will improve the future of my family and yours for many years to come. Sorry for the long introduction, but I feel that it is important to know a little about my background before I delve into this topic.

Enjoy the book,

Dan O.

What Are Stem Cells?

Stem cell, noun, BIOLOGY; plural noun: stem cells - An undifferentiated cell of a multicellular organism that is capable of giving rise indefinitely to more cells of the same type, and from which certain other kinds of cells arise by differentiation.

I was recently watching an episode of *Doctor Who*, the British Sci-Fi show, where they used miraculous microscopic repair robots that were programmed to repair and grow tissue, perfectly matched to the person's body based on their DNA.

I laughed. Not because it's science fiction, but because that's exactly what we already have in our body, our STEM CELLS.

We're using stem cells today to do exactly that. The key is figuring out where to get them from and how to make them do what we want them to do. People have been harvesting and moving tissue around to different parts of the body for many years now.

We're finally able to harvest these tiny little robots and move them to areas where we can use them instead of just storing them without benefit. Read on and understand that we are on the edge of the most incredible advance in medical technology by harnessing a blend of genetics, medicine and Mother Nature.

Chapter One: Buzz Word

Stem cells seem to be the medical buzz word of late and for good reason.

This treatment isn't just for celebrities and professional athletes anymore nor should it be viewed as immoral due to the advances in this technology.

Not too long ago people would travel to Germany, Russia or even Mexico to receive experimental treatments and even some treatments that are currently banned such as Fetal Stem Cells from aborted fetuses, but that is no longer the gold standard.

I think this issue is one of the biggest misunderstandings about stem cells among the general public. I can relate to both sides of the argument.

However, moral and personal beliefs should no longer be an issue because there are plenty of other types of stem cells that work just as well if not better than fetal stem cells. Fear not. We are not talking about killing fetuses or babies to grow stem cells for ourselves.

This book is about **non-embryonic stem cell transplantation**, so read on.

Aside from the embryonic stem cell issue, it's hard for a non-medical person to filter through the plethora of information there is about stem cells from the media, scientific journals and the internet.

You may also wonder about the different types of regenerative procedures such as PRP (Platelet Rich Protein) or Amniotic fluid therapy and why the price difference.

The goal of this book is to provide you with basic information about each of the alternatives and why you might choose one over the other for specific conditions. Once you have that data you should be able to make a decision that is right for you.

Our personal belief is that stem cell transplantation is the future of medicine. It's hard to be a skeptic when you have seen countless miracles unfold right before your eyes.

The problem that most physicians have with the new field of stem cell transplantation is that they are unfamiliar with it. It wasn't taught in medical school and most physicians don't have large pharmaceutical companies behind them funding study after study.

The reason why large private companies haven't been performing study after study is because running these will cost millions of dollars. I have personal knowledge of this since I have assisted in studies in graduate school and currently I am in the process of getting a basic device through the FDA which will still cost the company I am working for millions of dollars just to bring a rubber tourniquet to the public.

The reason why these large companies will invest millions of dollars of capital to bring a medication or device to the public is because they will hold a patent on it for about 20 years. This means no one else can make the same product for that time period.

If the device or medication is a success it means there are millions and possibly billions of dollars to be made during that 20 years.

Lipitor, a cholesterol medication, grossed $12.9 billion in 2006 during its peak and has grossed multiple billions every year after that as well.

Obviously, this was a grand slam for Pfizer - not all patents can make money like this. But this is the exact reason why someone is willing to risk everything and invest millions in studies to get a device or medication to the public.

To get a patent you need to make something that is 100% reproducible and it cannot be natural or naturally occurring. For example, no one gets to patent air and water and then charge you for its use.

Therefore stem cells are difficult to patent because they are natural. The exception to this is genetically modified cultured stem cell lines, which you can patent.

Your stem cells are slightly different than mine, along with my next patient's stem cells which is why there are virtually no patented stem cells.

Without the possibility of patenting, and the possibility of profit, there are fewer people willing to invest millions in studies just to prove that this is the best thing since sliced bread.

Since studies take millions of dollars, the founders of our network, **The Cell Surgical**

Network, have started a "patient funded research program."

Let me explain this a little; when a procedure is completed on a patient in our network, data about the results are published on our network database so we can determine what techniques, doses and procedures will provide the best outcomes in future treatment.

Over the years more and more data will be compiled and eventually more and more studies will be published.

This research is funded by patients paying for procedures and physicians recording that data with the goal of eventually making stem cells part of the standard of care which will be taught in medical schools.

We want this to become available for everyone and we want the process standardized so that a patient in California will receive the same protocol as someone in New York as well as Japan or Australia.

Imagine opting to have some of your very own stem cells injected into your arthritic back to heal your back which could reduce or eliminate your back pain? The same could be done for your shoulder, hip, knees, ankles or even other diseases.

Imagine using your own body to repair diseased organs, heal broken bones, damaged cartilage or torn tendons.

Imagine using this to treat neurological diseases like multiple sclerosis, Parkinson's, dementia, Alzheimer's and more.

The possibilities in the future could be limitless. Many of these diseases are even being treated with stem cells today.

Specific details about **autologous** (from your own body back to yourself) **fat derived stem cell transplant** will be mentioned later in the book, but the beauty of the protocol we currently are following is that a person can have this all done on the same day in about three hours at the office with very little downtime or risk of disease transmission or infection.

Physicians in the stem cell network have done over 4000 procedures without any major complication!

That's an amazing safety record and success rate. Think about your common hip replacement. How many people do you know who have had one of those? How often do you hear about someone complaining about a failure from a hip replacement?

Complications from a hip replacement varies by practitioner and Center but can be as high as 5%.

The stem cell protocol and technique that we advocate at this point has a 95 out of 100 case *success* rate and the Cell Surgical Network has done over 4000 of these transplants without a single serious complication.

When considering any new or old medical procedure, one must always consider the risks involved versus the potential benefits. With a track record like this one, it's hard to ignore this technology.

Now that we have discussed some of the basics, let's talk about the science of stem cells.

Chapter Two: Stem Cell Basics

The body is comprised of many organs and tissues, all of which function collectively as a cohesive unit to allow the body and each of its many components to properly work together.

The fundamental biological unit within the body is the cell. There are many different types of cells found in various tissues throughout the body.

Many of these cells are specialized into specific forms and types of cells, designed to carry out a range of particular functions, each with unique properties.

There are some cells, however, that are undifferentiated, and are not specialized into specific types. These cells are called stem cells, and these unspecialized cells undergo maturation to and can form more of their own kind.

These particular cells consist of growth factors along with essentially blank templates, such that stem cells can be transformed into various specific types, but no specialization has yet taken place when cells remain as stem cells.

Stem cell research has a long and rich history with various branches in medicinal applications for humans, as well as animals. The terminology of stem cells seems to have been coined between the 1860s and the 1880s, with German biologist Ernst Haeckel first doing so in 1868.

This was before William Sedgwick followed suit nearly two decades later in 1886. For almost a decade and a half since the terminology for a stem cell was first developed, scientists have worked tirelessly to try to uncover the secrets hidden behind these multipotent (means they can turn into different types of cells) and incredibly versatile cells.

It has been known for a long time that their potential use greatly outweighed their current status as useful tools in medicine and science, but the results are still continuing to approach the potential that has been known for some time.

The method used in our clinic utilizes stem cells derived from adipose (fat tissue) which is non-embryonic, non-fetal and autologous (taken from your body).

Embryonic stem cells have been hailed by the media in the past for their pluripotent property which means they can turn into any type of cell.

These cells come from embryonic development stage where this cell has the ability to make any tissue in your body, unlike adult stem cells which are multipotent. However, studies are beginning to show that adult stems cells from areas such as fat and bone marrow may be better suited for adult treatment because there is no risk of forming teratomas (a type of cancerous growth).

Embryonic cells are designed to grow a human being and have an extremely rapid growth process that has great potential but also carries a small amount of risk.

Adipose derived stem cells are NOT pluripotent (they are multipotent) but have enough capability to differentiate and heal damaged tissue for most adult cells. Fat stem cells have been documented to differentiate into nerve cells, tendon, ligament, discs, cartilage, muscle, etc.

Chapter Three: Stem Cell Basics Part II

Definition review: A stem cell is an undifferentiated cell that can differentiate (turn into) a specific type of cell and also has the capability to replicate.

This may not sound that impressive, but I assure you stem cells are the future of healthcare. These cells when activated they can turn into another type of cell and replicate over and over again until the damaged tissue is repaired.

Stem cells perform these actions based on signals from growth factors in the damaged tissue.

The forms of stem cells most people think of are embryonic stem cells from the fetus but that is only one source, which we mentioned in the introduction. The new types of stem cells that most practices are using are adult mesenchymal stem cells.

Remember that embryonic stem cells can turn into any type of tissue in the whole body, since we originated from that type of cell, and without that ability you wouldn't be here today.

Because they are gathered from aborted fetuses their use will carry certain philosophical and moral opposition by some.

The overall safety of this procedure is high but there is a small chance that the cells could turn into tumor cells because of their rapid growth process. There is also potential risk because this tissue is not from your own body and this could lead to unforeseen problems in the future.

Adult mesenchymal stem cells are found all over the body in your bone marrow and fat. Both can turn into most types of tissue in the body, but they are much safer to use than embryonic stem cells and the moral or ethical issues do not apply to this type of stem cell.

There is also no risk of rejection since the procedure uses autologous cells, which means they come from your own body and this also reduces the risk of bacterial or viral infections since the tissue is immediately returned to the body after the stem cells are isolated and activated.

These adult mesenchymal stem cells or adult stem cells (ASC) can form bone, cartilage, muscle, nerves, blood vessels, connective tissue and fat. These are called mesenchymal stem cells because they come from the mesodermal layer of your own partially developed embryo. That is why

ASC from this area works extremely well for most medical conditions. These cells have the ability to develop into any of the above tissues.

We will discuss this in further detail later but consider the power of a simple medical procedure that could make things like knee-replacement surgery unnecessary by simply regrowing the lost cartilage in the knee.

See the tissue model below of ASC from fat turning into other types of cells.

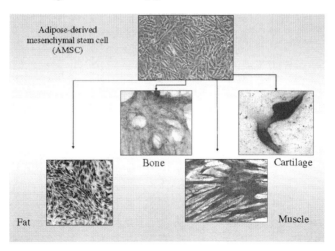

Chapter Four: How Do Stem Cells Work?

How Do Stem Cells Know What To Fix?

Your body is quite amazing. Stem cells have a homing property to specifically target injured cells.

Those damaged tissues will release cytokine signals that will draw in stem cells and other types of healing cells to help repair the cells.

Cytokines are specific signal proteins that are the way the body sends homing beacons or instructions to incoming cells and proteins.

These cytokines are bound to receptors and send instructions to cells so they know what to do.

The stem cells, having bound to the cytokine signals, will then start repairing the damaged tissue because of these repair request signals.

Growth factors are cytokines that are made up of amino acids that will literally provide instructions to the stem cells on what tasks they need to perform or what type of cell they need to turn into in order to repair the damaged cells.

They are naturally produced and have been used in many new age cosmetic products. They have also been used in orthopedic practices to increase healing speed using the growth factors in platelet rich protein (PRP) produced from your blood.

We will speak more about growth factors in a later chapter because they can be a viable alternative for many conditions at a fraction of the cost of stem cells.

Adult Mesenchymal Stem Cells

The current process that we advocate uses adult mesenchymal stem cells that are procured from your body fat using a minor liposuction procedure.

We utilize the layer of stromal vascular fraction (SVF) which will also contain macrophages, t-regulatory cells, endothelial cells, red blood cells, growth factors and micelles.

The adult adipose derived stem cells will remain dormant until they witness some tissue injury and receive signals from growth factors to activate them into functioning stem cells.

Adult mesenchymal stem cells have been successfully gathered from bone marrow but there are a few problems with that model.

Bone Marrow Harvesting

Bone marrow has a much lower quantity of stem cells present in the tissue. The stem cell count in bone marrow will be suppressed by chronic illness and will also decrease in numbers with age. The benefit of isolating stem cells from fat compared to bone marrow is that stem cells from fat do not significantly decrease with age or chronic disease.

Unfortunately for some patients who seek out stem cell therapy using bone marrow, they do not realize this until they find that the procedure didn't work as well as they hoped.

Using bone marrow can be very effective for younger individuals, but most of our patients who seek out stem cell treatment are either older and suffer from degenerative conditions or they have a chronic disease that would decrease the stem cell count in their bone marrow.

For this reason we opted to use fat over bone marrow for our ASC source at Desert Medical Care and Wellness.

Take a look at the graph below of stem cell counts from bone marrow and it isn't hard to see why bone marrow is a poor source for adult mesenchymal stem cells.

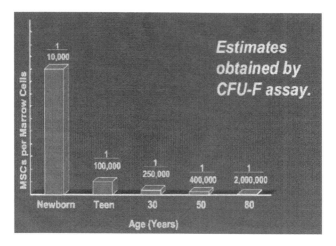

In your bone marrow at birth you will have 1 out of every 10,000 cells in your body made of stem cells.

By the time you are 50 years old, you will have 1 out of every 400,000 and by the age of 80 you will only have 1 out of 2,000,000, which is dismal at best.

This last figure will typically lead to about 60 to 600 stem/progenitor cells per ml.

whereas fat will contain 500,000 to 1,400,000 stem/progenitor cells per ml. (which is much more bang for your buck).

Note progenitor cells will have many qualities of stem cells except they cannot replicate as many times or differentiate into as many types of cells - they are descendants of stem cells and can only differentiate into certain types of cells.

Fat is made up of adipocytes and pre-adipocytes. Pre-adipocytes can multiply into additional fat cells (adipocytes) when challenged by an increase in caloric intake.

Believe it or not this is a survival mechanism no matter how unsightly it may make one look.

If your weight remains stable, these pre-adipocytes will remain dormant until a fat cell dies, which is when they will activate and turn into a new fat cell.

These pre-adipocytes, when separated from the fat and collagen, are the same as mesenchymal stem cells, which is why scientists and physicians are so excited with this very recent discovery.

Chapter Five: Will Stem Cell Treatment Make My Cartilage Look Different On An X-Ray & How Do You Know Where To Treat?

Take a look at this x-ray:

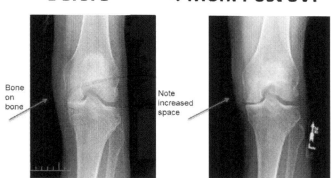

Before   **4 Mon. Post SVF**

Bone on bone

Note increased space

Some patients may have a visible change on their x-rays like the image shown above but not everyone will have a visible change after one treatment.

However, most will have a decrease or elimination of their pain after one treatment. In fact, most orthopedic conditions will have between a 70-90% improvement rate within a year of the treatment.

Some patients state they feel better within a week, most within a few months and some take an entire year. There hasn't been enough data on why some people improve faster than others, but there are studies about stem cell growth in a petri dish that have shown increased production of stem cells.

A petri dish is where we grow stem cells in the lab outside of a living organism and do not necessarily translate into the same behavior inside a human being.

How Do You Know Where to Treat ?

Over the next decade we will know more and more about what stem cells will be able to create and we will be able to design specific cells for certain treatments.

Eventually, as this subject is better understood, laws will allow us to grow and culture your own cells prior to deployment. Protocols will work better with different conditions but the good thing is that there has been nothing dangerous about the treatments so far.

In our practice we have primarily used adult stem cells to repair age or trauma related joint damage, which are our most common types of patients in our practice.

There are plenty of cases of autoimmune diseases that have been treated successfully with stem cells, but our practice deals primarily with pain patients. This is one of our treatment programs for pain conditions.

Knowing where to inject for a hip or a knee may be pretty easy for me, but with spinal injections there are too many options to just guess based on an MRI or x-ray, which is why we use MRIs with a radioactive dye that is injected which will clearly be shown on the image here.

This is an excellent alternative compared to the traditional MRI without contrast that will only show all of the structures, but not necessarily the area of injury, which is ultimately the area that needs immediate treatment. Notice on this MRI on the right it will show a bright spot on the L4/5 disc, indicative of a bulge and tear in the disc. The procedure to deliver stem cells in this area will be almost identical to an epidural injection except the medication is swapped out for stem cells in our case.

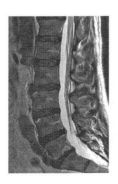 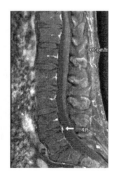

What About Neurological Conditions?

Since these stem cells can turn into nerve cells, there are cases of neurological diseases such as Parkinson's disease, strokes and demyelinating conditions that have shown improvement.

This is not a panacea nor is this a cure for these conditions but some of the outcomes have been very favorable with very little downside other than it potentially not working. As options go this is better than surgery or certain side effects of medications for these conditions. Especially since it can be tried virtually risk-free.

What Other Conditions Can Stem Cells Be Used For?

Stem cells can be used to treat a very wide range of conditions such as:

- Orthopedic conditions
- Degenerative conditions
- Cardiac conditions
- Pulmonary conditions

- Autoimmune conditions
- Urology
- Neurology
- Ophthalmology
- Cosmetic surgery

Within the Stem Cell Network there are different specialists that we utilize for certain procedures. For example our practice will do most of these procedures except for certain urological injections, brain injections and a few others because it is not our expertise.

Many of these hard to reach areas only require an IV drip of stem cells which is why we can treat many of these conditions. Specialized delivery of the stem cells into the eye requires a surgical ophthalmologist for deployment into the eye if needed.

Chapter Six: What Is The Process For Adipose Derived Stem Cell Treatment?

The Process

We use a closed sterile surgical system for SVF production (stromal vascular fraction – see Chapter 4 for a reminder). This means that the cells are not exposed to the environment prior to deployment into the body. This virtually eliminates the chance of contamination.

There are standard pre-operative protocols prior to the procedure like any minor surgery. Patients are asked to report any infections, surgeries, dental procedures at least 1 month prior to the procedure and 5 days prior they are asked to consider stopping their blood thinners. This is up to the surgeon and blood loss is absolutely minimal due to the minor incision made for the procedure.

The medications that are currently considered as blood thinning medications are: aspirin, Aggrenox, Coumadin, heparin, Lovenox, Plavix and Xarelto.

There is no restriction regarding the use of anti-inflammatories before or after the procedure, but some orthopedic surgeons and other regenerative protocols suggest that you stop these prior to and for a short time after the procedure.

Corticosteroid (cortisone) injections into the joint probably do not affect the SVF therapy, but to be safe we suggest that the stem cells be injected at least 1 month after the injection into that joint.

The day of the procedure, you will shower prior to the procedure and wash all of your areas thoroughly and wear loose, comfortable clothing that can easily fit over a surgical wrap.

There are no dietary restrictions before or after the procedure, however alcohol should not be consumed 8 hours prior to the procedure and your last meal before the procedure should be a light one rather than a heavy one in case you get nervous.

After the procedure we do not have any study that supports a specific type of diet, but common sense would suggest that a healthy diet with fresh vegetables, fruit, healthy protein, healthy fats and whole grains is better for anyone.

In the lab, stem cells grow faster with a nitric oxide product that improves circulation and this is offered to our patients, but we haven't had a study that shows that this improves our outcomes in humans and only in a petri dish at this point (petri dish is when we grow stem cells in a lab).

The area of fat that is typically used is the posterior flank or the "love handle" because of its ease of access, vascularity and the fact there are no major organs or possible hernias in that area.

If someone is extremely thin, we can typically find some fat near the buttocks as well.

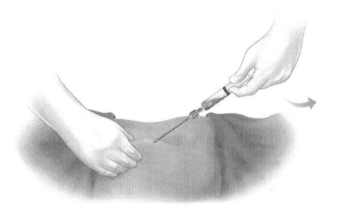

The amount of adipose fat tissue that is used to treat 2-3 areas is typically 50 cc or 1.7 ounces, which is not very much at all.

In fact, many patients jokingly even suggest that while we have them locally anesthetized, we pull out much more than that - but that's about as far as it goes.

The incision is so small that you will barely be able to see it in this photo, but I have inserted a picture of it so you can see how tiny it actually is.

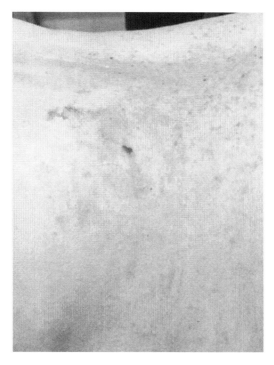

Afterwards, this area is cleaned up, sterilized again and covered with a dressing to absorb any leakage of the aesthetic fluid and blood. Finally, a piece of rubber foam is placed where the fat was harvested and a compression dressing is put on for 1-2 days to help smooth out the fat.

Then the process of isolating the stem cells begins. This part is very technical but does not take long. We will have your finished product after 90 minutes of work, which will be approximately 10 cubic centimeters (cc) of SVF, also known as liquid gold.

Each cc of this SVF will contain between 500,000-1,400,000 stem cells, which means you will have between 5-14 million stem cells per 10 ccs of SVF. Remember bone marrow will only have 60-600 stem cells per cc, which is obviously much less than SVF from fat.

Once you have this "liquid gold" you can either inject it into the affected area of the body and/or use an intravenous (IV) deployment.

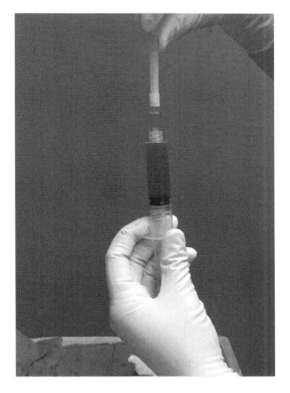

We typically will utilize both since most of our patients will have multiple problems, including spinal and extremity problems, along with other internal problems. Remember that the adult stem cells get activated when they find areas of tissue damage, which means that even an IV deployment will find areas of tissue damage.

All joint injections require an x-ray, which is done prior to the procedure and the needle is guided under ultrasound for all non-spinal joints and CT or fluoroscopy guidance for any spinal injections.

These are standard procedures taught in any medical specialty program and these devices are used to visualize important structures such as nerves, arteries and tendons that you will want to avoid when injecting.

Although this requires skill, in our office we provide these types of injections on a daily basis with regular medications so this is done within a few minutes and performed precisely.

Afterwards you should NOT engage in any strenuous activity, heavy lifting or athletics for a period of several days and there will be bruising where the liposuction took place. Driving home will not be an issue since there was only local aesthetic used during this procedure. If there is any discomfort, your doctor, who performed the procedure, will recommend an over the counter pain reliever and some ice.

Chapter Seven: Cells on Ice and the Future of Medicine?

Imagine that you were just playing a game of tennis and heard a pop in your knee and found out that your tore a tendon, or maybe you just have a chronic condition that eats away at your body like Rheumatoid Arthritis or maybe you just had a stroke and damaged your brain.

Imagine being able to treat all of these conditions with your very own cells made from your DNA to match your body.

This is a growing field called Bio-Insurance, which is where a facility will store your own cells for potential treatment of chronic diseases that you do not have yet. There already is a growing field of research of stem cell cancer treatments and there have been many successful cases of treating traumatic brain injury after an accident or stroke when treated within the ideal window of time.

Some of these treatments do not require a physician because the cell surgery is complete and the treatment only requires a nurse to hook up an IV cocktail bag while you sit and read a good book for 30 minutes.

The cells will target areas of inflammation and disease which is why this is great for chronic inflammatory conditions like Rheumatoid Arthritis and other auto-immune diseases.

Our bodies make trillions of stem cells over time but as we age these cells are replenished at a slower rate and eventually parts of your body start to break down.

This could lead to organ failure, tissue failure, joint failure or even failure of your nerves (which includes your brain).

If you wish to store your stem cells, it only requires a few simple steps.

First, you will have a blood test clearing you for infectious disease. Second, we will simply pull out an additional ounce of fat during our liposuction procedure. Third, we ship it to the storage facility overnight in a cryo-container which will freeze the cells as they are shipped.

Cells are stored at an FDA approved tissue storing facility which stores these cells at minus 190 degrees Celsius in liquid nitrogen. This process has been in use for years to store sperm, eggs, embryos and, more recently, umbilical cord blood and tissue.

We call this bio-insurance because you are banking this before you need it, just like insurance. I'm sure when you purchase car insurance you do not plan on getting in an auto accident, but that's why they are called accidents.

The best part about this is that you are using your own cells, with your own DNA, which mitigates any chance of an allergic reaction or disease transmission.

Chapter Eight: What Are PRP & Placental Derived Amniotic Fluid Used For?

Currently, many arthritic and degenerative conditions are being treated with stem cell applications but there are other less expensive alternatives to stem cells, in particular, amniotic fluid injections.

Amniotic fluid is rich in growth factors and has stem cell qualities to it. Amniotic fluid injections can be done at a fraction of the cost of real adult stem cells without any surgical harvesting procedure involved.

After having a close look at all the various amniotic fluid products on the market today, we chose to provide Placental Derived Amnion (PDA). PDA is the absolute closest product on the market to a "true" 361 tissue graft product. Just like our autologous stem cell product – less manipulation is better (as is often the case in medicine and many other disciplines as well).

Our amniotic fluid product is an acellular cocktail of growth factors, peptides and cytokines. It's harvested aseptically from planned cesareans and then processed immediately via centrifugation, followed by a stepped down freezing process.

No babies or fetuses are harmed in this process. It is harvested from fluid that is normally thrown away.

During the centrifugation process, all cellular material is removed and that's why this product is the most sterile on the market at 10^{-6} (1000 times more sterile than surgical instruments).

After that, the fluid is loaded into syringes and frozen. It's a simple fluid processing without denaturing cells via dehydration, powderization or mincing, which greatly reduces bioactivity.

Since bioactivity reduction is of course not ideal in these situations, we avoid that dilemma by the careful use of the procedures necessary to achieve the best possible results.

As well, there is no chorion product in our fluid, further serving to highlight the reasons why we offer the best and most effective option relative to our competitors.

In terms of where PDA fits into the treatment continuum, this would be a replacement for PRP for older patients (platelets decrease in number as we age).

It is also a replacement for patients that would traditionally be a "scratch" for an autologous regenerative therapy due an autoimmune disease like RA or perhaps a disease that affects healing like diabetes, just to name a few.

At the end of the day, autologous growth factor treatments like PRP are patient driven and results vary from person to person, device to device.

Amniotic fluid removes that patient variability and ensures a consistent level of bio-active growth factors at time of injection.

Once released the 120+ growth factors begin to recruit other endogenous regenerative cells and stem cells into the micro environment they are deployed in – regardless of the patient's overall health. Simply put, amniotic fluid helped bridge the gap so that anybody can utilize regenerative medicine no matter what their health history dictates.

The treatment using amniotic fluid simply involves the injection of it into the joint or tendons as needed. This will be done guided under ultrasound or fluoroscopy to visualize the needle moving to the area of injury.

Platelet Rich Protein (PRP)

Another growth factor treatment that has been performed for well over a decade is the use of growth factors out of your own blood known as **Platelet Rich Protein** or Platelet Rich Plasma Therapy (PRP), a non-surgical treatment for soft tissue injuries and joint pain.

PRP stimulates the body's natural healing forces, which is an excellent way of getting the body to work in the favor of the patient, rather than in opposition to the patient.

Often a patient using PRP will be able to avoid more invasive procedures such as surgery. If surgery is not an option, or a less invasive procedure is simply desired, PRP is a viable option with a lesser risk and shorter recovery time in many cases.

Chronic soft tissue injuries can be treated with PRP as an alternative to steroids. The beauty of PRP is that it has the ability to offer these alternatives in a safe and convenient package.

What Is PRP?

PRP, or Platelet Rich Plasma, is a substance made from your own blood to trigger healing. Any time you can harness the power of your own body and the blood it contains to heal yourself, that is a definite bonus.

Platelet Rich Plasma Therapy is a relatively simple, non-surgical treatment for joint injuries and arthritis. It merges cutting-edge technology with the body's natural ability to heal itself. It is also perfectly typed and cross matched to your body because it comes from your own body.

The PRP is a concentration of platelets, which can jump-start healing. Platelets contain packets of growth hormones and cytokines that tell the tissues to increase rebuilding in order to enhance healing.

When PRP is injected into the damaged area, it stimulates a mild inflammatory response, which triggers the healing cascade. This leads to restored blood flow, new cell growth, and tissue regeneration. This may ultimately result in faster healing of soft tissue injuries.

Safer, more effective procedures with shorter down times and more rapid recovery are the result of these advanced procedures, and patients reap the benefits when they select these options over more invasive surgical procedures.

Where does PRP come from?

A sample of blood is taken from a vein in a patient's arm under sterile conditions. The blood is then be placed in a centrifuge, which is a device that spins the blood down to distinct layers based on density.

This helps to separate the blood cells from the plasma, and allows concentration of the platelets. The layers can then be extracted and harvested for use.

This purified sample of platelets increases healing growth factors approximately six to eight times greater than normal. Its simple techniques like these that make these types of procedures so effective and efficient.

The preparation takes as little as 15 minutes. The finished PRP product is then available for injection into the injured joint or tendon under ultrasound guidance.

Because PRP is prepared from your own blood, there is no concern for rejection or disease transmission. In fact, PRP contains a high concentration of white blood cells, which helps to fight infection.

So rather than risk infection with the complications of potentially dangerous surgeries, this option actually serves to decrease the chances of an infection taking place.

What are the potential benefits?

PRP enhances your healing potential. It has proven to often be an effective and natural alternative to steroid injections.

Patients can see a significant improvement in symptoms as well as a remarkable return of function. This may eliminate the need for more aggressive treatments such as long-term medication or surgery.

Again, these positive aspects are certainly pros that point to the tremendous benefits of using procedures like PRP over surgical alternatives.

What Can I Expect During My Treatment?

You will visit with the doctor, who will ask about your medical history and give you a brief exam to determine that you are a good candidate for PRP therapy. If it's a good fit with your goals, we will obtain the blood sample and prepare the PRP.

The doctor will examine the area to be treated, sterilely prepare it, and apply numbing medicine. Typically, using ultrasound guidance, the PRP will be gently injected into the injured area and joint support tissues.

After your treatment, you will stay for a 30-minute observation period. At checkout, you will schedule a follow-up appointment and we will review discharge instructions to ensure you remain safe, comfortable, and healthy. The process may be repeated one to two times over a six to 16 week period.

What Can I Expect After the PRP Treatment?

You may have mild to moderate discomfort which may last up to a week. There may be temporary worsening of symptoms due to a stimulation of the inflammatory response, which is necessary for healing.

Your doctor will instruct you in the use of ice, elevation, reduced activity, and analgesic medications for comfort while the PRP is initiating healing.

Additionally, physical therapy or a therapeutic exercise program will be prescribed in an effort to further facilitate your healing and advance your recovery towards the optimal point in the shortest possible amount of time.

What Should I Do When I Get Home Following the Procedure?

Because Platelet Rich Plasma releases growth factors, it is important to not disturb the area of injection for at least 48 hours. We ask that you refrain from activities other than necessary walking or driving in order to receive the maximum benefit of the PRP growth factor stimulation.

It is helpful if you can be sedentary for 48 hours, and refrain from any vigorous activity for up to 2 weeks following each procedure.

What Medications Can I Take?

Please do not take any anti-inflammatory medications such as Ibuprofen, Aleve, Motrin or Aspirin. You may take Tylenol or you may be prescribed an appropriate analgesic, if necessary.

If you are on an 81-mg daily dose of aspirin for cardiovascular reasons, please do not take it within the first 48 hours.

PRP is a very effective non-stem cell therapy that still allows patients to avoid the use of invasive surgical procedures, and the pros of this approach far outweigh the cons.

PRP is a great alternative to try for mild to moderate degenerative conditions because of its low cost compared to all of the other options I mentioned earlier.

There are no stem cells in this protocol, but the blood is fairly simple to process, it is autologous (your own cells) so there is no chance of rejection and we use an airless system, which virtually eliminates any chance of an infection.

One factor to consider for PRP is the health of the individual because growth factors will decrease in your blood as you age.

They will decrease based on your health, which is something to consider when comparing this to amnion injections.

Amniotic fluid will have significantly more in the way of healing properties compared to PRP, but it will cost more than double the price.

There are many things to consider when contemplating whether surgery or stem cell treatment or something else is best for a certain ailment.

Factors such as cost, safety, effectiveness, and recovery time should all be taken into account to ensure that the most suitable decision is reached.

Sometimes surgery can be avoided entirely, and the results from these situations are becoming increasingly favorable as modern science provides techniques that are becoming better and better in the medical realm.

Chapter Nine: What Else Can You Do With Growth Factors?

There are various companies that will now engineer growth factors for specific cosmetic conditions such as skin, vaginal rejuvenation and hair growth. Companies can specifically engineer these cosmetic products, but cannot do the same for stem cells.

The market leader in this area comes from one of our network's affiliate doctors, Dr. Ahmed Al-Qahtani of AQ Solutions.

For cosmetic purposes we currently only carry their product line because no other company has achieved results that are comparable to AQ in this category.

GF-technology refers to AQ's advanced, cutting edge methods of producing human growth factors and utilizing them in topical skin care products.

Growth factors (GF) are found in many different cell types in the human body. They are a group of specialized proteins with many functions, the most important being the activation of cellular proliferation and differentiation.

Growth factors turn essential cellular activities "on" and "off," and they play a role in increasing cell production, cell division, blood vessel production, and collagen and elastin production.

In recent decades, scientific research into GF biological functions has shown that medical GF-technology is related to resolving many cell developmental diseases.

What Can You Do With Growth Factors?

But GF-technology has many other applications to human health and can also help people achieve a more youthful and vibrant look without expensive plastic surgery or Botox treatments.

It can even help people obtain healthy, fuller-looking hair without the side effects of drugs.

Growth factors are vital to maintaining a youthful appearance. The skin and scalp contain multiple growth factors that regulate natural cellular renewal and damage repair processes to keep skin healthy and to maintain a normal hair growth cycle.

These growth factors are responsible for helping to reverse the visible effects of chronological aging and premature aging due to environmental factors.

The consequences of environmental exposure and the normal processes of aging lead to excessive free radical damage of skin and scalp cellular components. This results in the breakdown of collagen and elastin networks in the dermis and produces the effect of visible facial aging.

This same type of damage eventually impairs growth factor function, so they are less able to repair oxidative damage, and the damage becomes permanent.

Advances in GF-technology are providing help for reversing the signs of aging. Growth factors can now be produced in a laboratory for topical use.

In multiple clinical studies, topically applied GF have been shown to reduce the signs of skin aging, including statistically significant reductions in fine lines and wrinkles and increases in dermal collagen synthesis.

GF-technology is also being used successfully for encouraging healthy hair growth, reducing the appearance of scars, supporting the skin during post-procedure healing, and shortening the healing time of burn wounds.

What Can You Do With Growth Factors?

The science of growth factors as an anti-aging skin technology moved forward a great deal through the work of scientists Stanley Cohen and Rita Levi-Montalcini, who were awarded the Nobel Prize in Medicine in 1986 for advancing understanding of the role of Epidermal Growth Factor (EGF) in cell biology.

Other researchers continued studying EGF, leading to current clinical applications of EGF for skin conditions and reversing the signs of aging. EGF is known to considerably increase skin cell regeneration, and studies have shown that it significantly aids in the healing of skin wounds.

Since the work of Cohen and Levi-Montalcini, scientific research has built a knowledge base of types and functions of other major GF, including TGF-b (Transforming Growth Factor), PDGF (Platelet Derived Growth Factor), GM-CSF (Granulocyte-Macrophage Colony-Stimulating Factor), and IL (Interleukins).

Medical research has found that GF can speed and improve healing when applied to areas of the human body damaged in surgery, burns, wounds, or accidents.

The mechanism behind the benefits is facilitation of changes at the cellular level to revert damaged cells to a younger state, healing the damaged skin in the process.

Some researchers wondered if the same GF-technology that was bringing such remarkable healing results to skin injuries could bring about cosmetic benefits as well. Scientists found that GF-technology had the potential to reverse the cell aging process, fade scars, improve healing, and renew the hair follicles on the scalp to help people with thinning hair.

GF-technology is now being shown to improve the appearance of aging and sun-damaged skin and to help restore normal hair growth. Cosmetic patents of early GF-technology were first issued in 1994.

What Can You Do With Growth Factors?

In 2001, two independent double-blind studies testing topical creams containing either natural or bio-engineered GF were presented to the Society of Investigative Dermatology.

The results were surprising—when applied to skin twice a day for four–six weeks, both types of creams produced better results than Botox! Each study showed significant increases in production of collagen, hyaluronic acid, elastin, fibroblasts, and epidermal thickness.

Now, AQ has made another major advance in GF-technology by developing unique serums for the skin and scalp that contain the ideal types and combinations of GF to produce maximum anti-aging and hair restoration results.

They have a great skin care product but here are a few of their unique products that definitely work well.

Here is information about the hair growth product:

Hair Solutions: Acts on the scalp to nourish and repair hair follicles, allowing for normal, healthy hair growth.

Scalp-specific growth factor combination stimulates hair follicle generation and new hair growth.

This treats thinning hair, hair loss, hardening of the scalp, and weak hair. This new GF-technology remedy effectively addresses hair loss at the source, by repairing damaged hair follicles and stimulating regeneration of active, new hair follicles.

The GF-technology utilized is the same remarkable technology behind the skin serums, but the growth factors in Advanced Hair Complex are carefully refined and selected for the special needs of the scalp.

Thinning hair is often caused by a scalp damaged by a dry climate, nutrition, stress, certain drugs, chlorine, and/or environmental exposure. Over many years, the skin of the scalp produces less growth factors and becomes less efficient at repairing damage.

Because of this, the condition of the scalp can eventually deteriorate to the point where it hardens (fibrosis) or hair follicles become miniaturized. In the case of fibrosis, hair is unable to grow through the hardened scalp.

Miniaturization renders the hair follicles unable to perform their normal growth cycle. Both conditions can lead to a cessation of hair production and the death of hair follicles.

Advanced Hair Complex is formulated to nourish hair follicles back to a state of ideal health with select growth factor proteins that are naturally present in healthy, young hair follicles.

This process allows for a normal hair growth cycle that leads to new hair growth and thicker, fuller-looking hair.

Stem cells lining the hair follicles are crucial for production of hair, and the GF-technology ingredients in this concentrated serum are selected to provide support to these stem cells, so hair can re-grow.

Advanced Hair Complex improves the overall condition of the scalp, rejuvenating damaged hair follicles and increasing circulation of nutrients for healthy hair.

The serum's action is enhanced by protective flower extracts, which help maintain cellular health and lustrous hair. The product has no greasy feel or unpleasant odor.

Another product they have remedies a problem that many post-menopausal women suffer from but do not talk about with their doctor, and that is vaginal dryness, decreased vaginal sensitivity and decrease in pleasure from intercourse.

The product is called VRS and it is for vaginal dryness and increasing sensitivity. It has been used very successfully and has been reported back as an "anti-aging" product in its own way.

VRS addresses the following:

- Relieving vaginal dryness and soothing irritation

- Improving elasticity, tightening and firming the vaginal walls

- Enhancing female sexual arousal and intercourse

- Rejuvenating vaginal function utilizing Growth Factor (GF) technology

VRS is a breakthrough solution for vaginal rejuvenation. Through Growth Factor technology, the VRS serum serves as part of the body's natural lubrication, which consists of thick fluid that is deposited to contact the walls encircling the vagina.

VRS rejuvenates the vagina by helping to restore the body's natural vaginal function. Further, VRS can help women achieve heightened vaginal sensations. VRS is formulated and designed to hydrate the interior vaginal walls and create a tightening effect, thus allowing more sensation and youthful resilience to an important part of the body, which is why some will say this product may be a female equivalent to Viagra for men.

If you have dark circles and bags under your eyes, we typically recommend the eye serum product. This is what AQ says about this product:

Eye serum lightens and tightens the eye area for a more youthful appearance with a highly concentrated formula containing a unique blend of new generation peptides and GF (growth factor)-technology.

Specially formulated and gentle enough for the eye area, Eye Serum promotes smoother, younger-looking skin.

It stimulates the skin's natural process of repair and rejuvenation by providing the biological elements that are present in young, healthy skin. The concentrated GF-technology blend stimulates collagen production for increased firmness, while several smoothing peptides help tighten and lift sagging skin.

Through activation of the skin's own damage repair processes, fine lines and wrinkles are smoothed. It increases micro-circulation and lightens the under-eye area, clearing up "bags" and dark circles.

The moisturizing formula supports the health of skin to maintain results and will not irritate even the most sensitive eyes. This pure, non-greasy serum has a clean smell and will not clog pores.

Conclusion

We've talked about many different keys to Regenerative Medicine and even touched on Physical Medicine for a brief moment. Just to recap, we learned about different types of procedures from cosmetic growth factors use to autologous growth factors from your blood used for pain relief.

We discussed what stem cell options there are in the world and the United States and what the difference is between adult and embryonic stem cells.

We discussed safety, low infection rate, results and even discussed procedure for adipose derived stem cells.

To conclude I'll leave you with the #1 secret for achieving great results which is taking action and becoming the ambassador of your own health.

You've already done that by picking up this book and reading this, which is better than 90% of the people out there, but information without action is useless.

As your condition progresses and gets worse the likelihood of you achieving optimal results from stem cells or growth factor treatment will decrease but that isn't to say you won't get results, because we have treated chronic lower back pain in 90 year old patients with great success.

That also doesn't mean you should leave it forever, doing something is better than nothing.

CONTACT INFORMATION:

I know it is hard to cram all of this information into this short book, but we tried. Honestly each case is different so the best thing to do at this point is to request a free consultation so we could inform you about your specific situation.

There is also more information, which is continuously updated, to be found at: http://stemcellrevolution.com

The best way you could reach us either at 760-777-8377 or 760-848-4999 and we can be found online at:

www.DesertMedicalCare.com .

During your office visit, you will have a one-on-one appointment with one of the doctors in our clinic. Please fill out your patient paperwork found at:

www.DesertMedicalCare.com

That will provide our team the information I need to make a recommendation. Your initial visit should take no more than 45 minutes, but this 45 minutes may change the rest of your life.

Once you have filled out the forms, just call 760-777-8377 to set up your free life changing appointment today.

NOTES

Index

Index

35150449R00059

Made in the USA
Columbia, SC
25 November 2018